3-25

Care of the Dying
A Clinical Handbook

Care of the Dying
A clinical handbook

Nigel C. H. Stott BSc FRCPEd MRCGP
Welsh National School of Medicine, Cardiff

Ilora G. Finlay MRCGP DCH DRCOG
Maryhill Health Centre, Glasgow

Nursing Adviser:
De'arne Goldie SRN DNS HV
St Columba's Hospice,
Edinburgh

Illustrated by
Adrian Shaw and Janice Sharp
Department of Medical Illustration and AudioVisual Services,
Welsh National School of Medicine

CHURCHILL LIVINGSTONE
EDINBURGH LONDON MELBOURNE AND NEW YORK 1984

CHURCHILL LIVINGSTONE
Medical Division of Longman Group Limited

Distributed in the United States of America by Churchill
Livingstone Inc., 1560 Broadway, New York, N.Y.
10036, and by associated companies, branches and
representatives throughout the world.

© Longman Group Limited 1984

First published 1984

ISBN 0 443 03160 6

British Library Cataloguing in Publication Data
Stott, Nigel C.H.
  Care of the dying.
  1. Terminal care
  I. Title   II. Finlay, Ilora G.
  362.1'75   R726.8

Library of Congress Cataloging in Publication Data
Stott, Nigel C. H. (Nigel Clement Halley), 1939–
  Care of the dying.
  1. Terminal care   I. Finlay, Ilora G.   II. Title.
R726.8.S746   1984   616'.029   84–5034

Printed in Hong Kong by
Wing King Tong Co Ltd.

Preface

During the past decade the care of the dying has begun to become a speciality, but it is also quite clear that most people will not be cared for in specialised terminal care units for personal, logistic or humanitarian reasons. Professor E. Wilkes and others, in the report of the Working Party on Terminal Care (DHSS Standing Medical Advisory Committee March 1980) concluded that 'the way forward is to encourage dissemination of the principles of terminal care throughout the health service . . .' (para. 4.1).

This book has been written to provide a concise handbook for those clinicians and nurses who need a ready reference manual. We believe that many patients will die more peacefully and gracefully if their terminal problems are approached in a systematic and compassionate way. The text has been kept to a minimum and we have used illustrations liberally in an attempt to highlight the human feelings in each problem as well as to portray some solutions in as succinct a way as possible.

Very few aspects of terminal care are truly specialised because the topic embraces almost every aspect of good clinical and nursing practice. For this reason we have approached care of the dying as general clinicians who face problems in the home as well as in hospital and we have made no attempt to include detailed specialist information or techniques which are relevant to a minority of patients. We gratefully acknowledge the inspiration and information which pioneers in the field of terminal care have shared with us. We share the enthusiasm of so many specialists and generalists who are re-discovering the importance of 'care' in clinical practice.

Currently approximately one-third of cancer patients die at home in Britain compared with two-thirds who die in other places (mostly hospitals) and this has been interpreted as a swing in society against care of the dying at home. Like many selected statistics, this cruelly underestimates the enormous workload which families, district nurses and general practitioners undertake for weeks, months or even years before the final entry of a patient as an in-patient, often less than two weeks before death. We hope that all who apply the principles in this book will honour both the carers and the regimes because the grief or anger of carers is often greater if they have not been valued and encouraged during the testing months before the death of a relative or friend. Care of the dying should be one of the ministries of hope and encouragement.

We wish particularly to acknowledge the following: Dr Richard Hillier, Dr Tom West, Professor Eric Wilkes, Dr Derek Doyle, Dr Thelma Bates, Dr Mary Baines, Dr Averil Stedeford, Dame Cicely Saunders, Professor Robert Harvard Davis, Dr Peter Griffiths, Dr Robert Twycross and the Oxford Course on Terminal Care, St Christopher's Hospice Course on Terminal Care for General Practitioners, The Multi-disciplinary Group for Care of the Dying in South Glamorgan, St David's Foundation Newport, Mrs Mary Stott, Dr Andrew Finlay.

Cardiff   N.C.H.S.
1984   I.G.F.

Contents

1

General approach

When you are dying it is difficult to forget a disease which seems so destructive. The problem also confronts physicians and it can modify clinical judgement adversely if death is always felt to be a failure. But death should be no failure if the carers are sound because it can be the beginning of new life or a peaceful finale. However, there is never room for complacency towards the end of life because fears, jealousy or resentments can cut away any hard-won ground and professional carers dare not be islands of expertise. Instead they must enjoy team-work and the demands of clinical problems which may straddle the whole of medical and nursing care. Relative, friend, volunteer, nurse, doctor, social worker, spiritual confidant or legal adviser — each one can help or hinder the peace which can be present at the end of mortal life and the wise clinician will give due recognition to all who care because they are strengthened by feeling valued.

Whenever a change in symptoms occurs, e.g. more pain, it is important to go back to first principles and ask 'why this has happened?' and 'what is the cause?'. Prescribing for the symptom can only be appropriate if the cause is assessed. This may seem a trite comment, but all too often vigorous symptom analysis is abandoned once a disease has been announced 'incurable'. Precision in care is just as important as precision in cure and three general aspects to care of the dying are our special concern:

1. The patient's problems (physical and emotional, social and spiritual).

2. The doctor's/nurse's attitudes, knowledge and skills.

3. Relatives' reticence and lack of confidence to use their own skills in the face of apparent professional expertise.

It is too easy for professional people to 'take over' from relatives and friends and to encourage lay carers to feel that their loved one is 'in the best hands away from home in hospice or hospital'. Sometimes this will be true but often it is not. Transfer of responsibility can seriously undermine the confidence of the lay-carers just when they need to feel involved or valued. Separation is always painful when loving relationships exist and so the following principles are worth remembering:

1. Honour both patients AND carers at all times and do nothing which will weaken the bonds of trust between them.

2. Build on what exists locally and don't undermine it even if it is second best (or you may end up with worse).

3. Never allow a hospital or hospice to become more important than the patient's home because home is where people usually want to spend their twilight months.

4. If peace and confidence are absent in the carers of the patient, you may be the wrong person to be in charge of this particular patient.

5. Fear of death is often greatest in those who have never felt bereavement. Relatives need constant encouragement to stay with the dying person and to be actively involved in their care — this is usually what the patient wants and it is the beginning of the process of working towards a healthy bereavement.

There is never 'no hope' — even the most extensive disease can undergo an unexpected/miraculous remission and, for many, hope is closely linked to peace about the future: the peace of mind that comes after a good fight is right for some, the peace that comes from leaving order behind is for others, the peace of spiritual confidence is a cherished goal for many.

These general points are, of course, central to the whole practice of modern primary health care and many were well rehearsed in the Alma Ata Declaration of the World Health Organization. Their relevance to death and dying simply reinforce their importance to society as a whole. In this little text we can focus on the end-phase of life, but, as primary physicians, we must see this as only part of a whole. Our nursing and spiritual colleagues have always supported this approach and it can now become strengthened by the advantages of modern symptom control together with more open mutual understanding with our patients.

2

Talking to patients and their families

Every experienced doctor or nurse grows to realise that patients assimilate information about themselves and their diseases at very variable rates. A few will want the A–Z spelt out, but most will absorb fragments of the truth over a period of days, weeks or months. Patients discuss the issues with family and friends and so the questions they ask are often those of their relations as much as their own. The clinician who understands this process of assimilation will realise that he/she is part of a continuing discourse and the biggest challenge is not what to say, but to listen carefully so the patient's questions, fears or doubts can be answered truthfully when they are ready to receive the information.

A dubious ethical situation arises when clinicians give relatives confidential information concerning a patient who is unaware of the diagnosis. This practice places an unfair burden on the family and often inhibits the normal process of enquiry which the patient and relatives pursue together. Genuine sharing of anything involves an honest relationship, hence sharing the burden of sorrow or worry can only occur normally when the family are functioning as a unit.

It is always hard for a clinician to impart painful information without feeling that he/she is dispensing hopelessness. However, there is always 'hope' because hope is a personal phenomenon which is generated in some people by a fight, in some by leaving order behind them, in some through the pursuit of remaining goals, in some through confidence in a spiritual future and in some because they have long ago come fully to terms with their own mortality.

The clinician seldom knows the values and deeper background of the patient so there is no alternative but to allow the patient and family together to consult on many occasions to discuss and discover the information they need.

The patient is bound to grieve (sometimes angrily) for his/her waning health and relatives often fear the changes they face. Allowing these feelings to be expressed verbally or non-verbally demands patience and understanding from those who are not emotionally involved, particularly as the same issues sometimes need to be repeated again and again before the patient and family come to terms with their futures.

3

Avoiding confusion over therapy and food

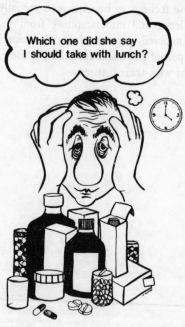

Which one did she say I should take with lunch?

Avoiding therapeutic confusion is only possible at home if the patient or relatives understand and control the treatment. A chart is a useful aid which improves co-operation because it encourages a routine by displaying the medication and its actions. Some patients will stand it on the mantelpiece or television for all to see and discuss, others are more reticent, but all are more likely to understand what is happening when medication charts are used.

		TIMES					
		morning		afternoon		night	
Clear medicine (Morphine for pain)	5 ml teaspoon	6	10	2	6	10	2
Blue medicine (Stemetil)	5 ml teaspoon	6	10	2	6	10	2
Maxolon	1 tablet	6		2		10	
Orange Medicine (Dorbanex Forte) for bowels	1 tblspoon					10	
Dexamethasone	2 tablets	6		2		10	

Medication chart

To determine the dosage interval it is vital to know the duration of action of all the drugs. This is frequently overlooked by hasty clinicians who, for example, have been known to prescribe dextromoramide (Palfium) b.d. for chronic pain. Page 8 illustrates how little pain relief could be expected from such a regime.

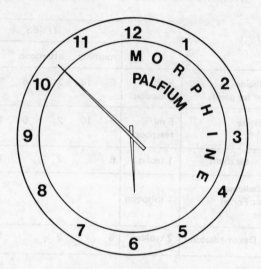

The half-life of each drug is important information which will determine the duration of action when metabolic processes are normal.

Simple dietary advice is also important, because insufficient intake of fluids, fibre or nutrients can result in unnecessary suffering and medication. Food symbolises love and communication within the home and eating can still give pleasure to many dying people. A little time with the patient and spouse or relative to work out what is enjoyable, practical and nutritionally desirable can give confidence to the carers who should continue to provide imaginative meals/drinks.

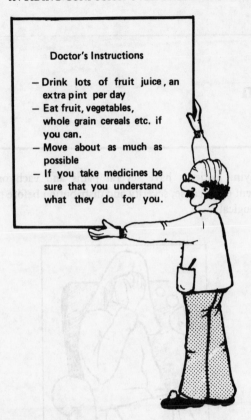

Doctor's Instructions

- Drink lots of fruit juice, an extra pint per day
- Eat fruit, vegetables, whole grain cereals etc. if you can.
- Move about as much as possible
- If you take medicines be sure that you understand what they do for you.

The aims of the patient are, for as long as possible:

1. Enjoyment of life.
2. Meeting nutritional (especially fluid) needs.
3. Maintenance of comfortable bowel function.
4. The social contact which comes with meals and over a cup of tea.

4

Pain

Most dying patients have several pains and each one needs assessment of its cause, severity and distribution before treatment can be logical.

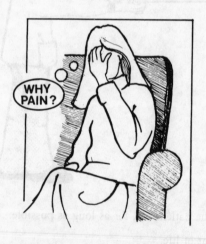

The cause of pain requires constant review. Many problems respond best to forms of treatment other than simple analgesics, e.g. nerve pressure pain, raised intracranial pressure, neuralgia, lymphoedema, infections or gastro-intestinal colic merit different forms of management which may reduce the analgesic requirements.

Understanding a patient's pain(s) is aided by involving the patient in the assessment. This is most easily done by discussing a body chart with the patient who can point to sites of pain and describe their characteristics (see figures on pp. 11 or 12). Frequently patients experience several different types of pain and each one may require a different therapeutic approach.

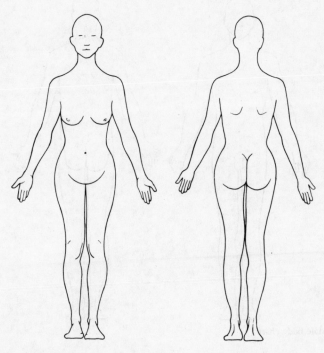

Female body chart

Weakened people are much more susceptible to pains from pressure areas, ligamentous sprains, myalgia, cramps, cystitis, constipation etc. and so the cause of the terminal illness must be seen as only one possible source of discomfort. The management of soft tissue and musculo-skeletal pains often hinges on nursing care, maintenance of mobility and physiotherapy. The pain threshold is also lowered by fear or anxiety or unhappiness.

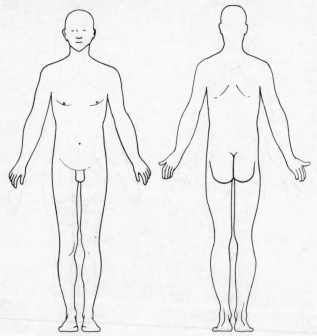

Male body chart

CONTROL OF PAIN

Only about 50 per cent of patients experience physical pain in their terminal illness but most patients will benefit from the application of certain principles which have been well worked out by pioneers in the hospice movement.

1. The nature of a person's distress can change from day to day because the disease is progressive and pain has physical, emotional, social and spiritual antecedents.

2. The doctor/nurse must not feel that death is a failure.

3. The patient and family will need help to articulate their fears or difficulties because coming to terms with impending death is a gradual process which is very painful for all concerned.

4. Many very simple and practical aids or sources of help are extremely important to the family and patient. The control of pain is not just a prescribing process.

5. The family and patient must always feel that a further source of help is available if their ability to cope begins to wane.

The practical application of these important principles is a massive challenge to all those concerned with care of the dying. Drug therapy can only benefit the patient fully if these general principles are also applied.

Choice of analgesics

Every analgesic must be given in adequate amounts and frequently enough to keep the patient essentially pain free. This can only be achieved if the clinician titrates the therapy up or down to achieve optimum control and is willing to review drug requirements constantly.

```
CLINICAL TARGET =
FREE FROM PAIN 24 HOURS A DAY
```

When changing analgesic or route of administration, the dose is determined by comparing their analgesic equivalence (see p. 15).

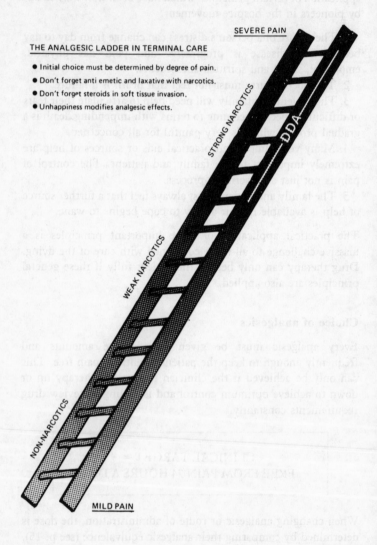

SEVERE PAIN

THE ANALGESIC LADDER IN TERMINAL CARE

- Initial choice must be determined by degree of pain.
- Don't forget anti emetic and laxative with narcotics.
- Don't forget steroids in soft tissue invasion.
- Unhappiness modifies analgesic effects.

DDA

STRONG NARCOTICS

WEAK NARCOTICS

NON-NARCOTICS

MILD PAIN

EXAMPLES ON THE ANALGESIC LADDER   (+ Morphine equivalence)

DIAMORPHINE INJECTIONS 4 hrly (1 mg ≡ 3 mg oral morphine)

MORPHINE ORALLY - as elixir 4 hrly (5 - 200 mg)
                    - as M.S.T. tablets, 12 hrly (dose : page 19)
        SUPPS - 10, 15, 20, 30 or 60 mg sizes.

PHENAZOCINE (Narphen) - sublingual tablet 6 hrly
                        (5 mg ≡ 15 mg morphine)

OXYCODONE SUPPS - (30 mg ≡ 15 mgs rectal morphine)

CODEINE DERIVATIVES - codeine phosphate 30 - 60 mg 4 hrly.
                          - in combination with aspirin or paracetamol
ASPIRIN with PAPAVERETUM effervescent tablets 4 hrly.

DEXTRO PROPOXYPHENE with PARACETAMOL   (Distalgesic)

SIMPLE ANALGESICS - ASPIRIN soluble or E.C.
                       - PARACETAMOL

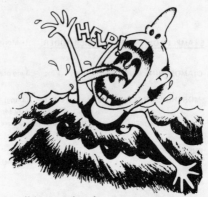

**Prescribing analgesics for terminal patients
on a p.r.n. basis is often like taking a drowning
man up for air and then pulling him down again**

To maintain blood levels and therefore pain control, it is often
better to disturb the sleeping patient for a dose (some patients can
sleep through the 2 a.m. dose but not all). Oral solutions should
be mixed at the bedside and any flavouring required can then be
added, e.g. Ribena or soda water.*

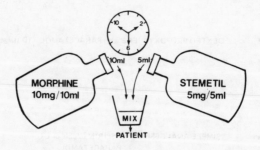

---

*Morphine slow-release tablets can maintain blood levels on a b.d. regime
(see p. 19).

Suggested prescription when starting oral morphine:

1. Morphine salt 10 mg

   water to 5 ml

   5 ml 4 hourly regularly

   250 ml = 500 mg morphine

2. Stemetil 5 mg/5 ml

   5 ml 8 hourly with morphine

   250 ml

3. Dorbanex Forte 10–20 ml daily

   500 ml

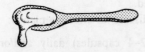 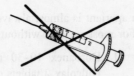

Use oral morphine if possible

**MORPHINE SHOULD NOT BE WITHHELD
FROM PATIENTS UNTIL PAIN IS SEVERE**

Problems with morphine

Tolerance

This does not develop significantly if the patient is given an adequate dose to remain pain-free. There is no reason why patients shouldn't remain on morphine for many months.

Sedation

It is worth warning the patient about temporary sedation which wears off in 2-3 days.

Dependence

Addiction does not develop if opiates are given for pain control. After another treatment to remove the pain, e.g. radiotherapy or nerve block, morphine can be tailed off over 2-3 days.

Respiratory Depression

The analgesic dose is lower than the depressant dose, so titrating up to the analgesic dose avoids respiratory depression.

Constipation

An aperient is almost always required.

For most patients without bowel disease an effective plan is:

1. Dorbanex 10-30 ml (or 2-4 capsules) daily and/or Dulcolax 2 tablets or suppository every 2nd-4th day,

with 2. an increased fluid intake, e.g. fruit juice,

with 3. increased fibre intake (if possible).

Nausea and vomiting

An antiemetic, e.g. prochlorperazine or haloperidol, should be given with the morphine from the beginning. Some patients can gradually cut it out after a week, but not all.

Why not Brompton cocktail instead?

Alcohol stings a sore mouth and cocaine causes hallucinations. If chlorpromazine is added it is very sedative. It is difficult to titrate away pain with a cocktail of fixed proportions because side effects are more likely.

Other forms of opiates

M.S.T. tablets (morphine slow-release tablets)

Morphine also comes as M.S.T. tablets in varying strengths and these can be used on a b.d. dosage as they are a slow release formulation (see p. 14).

The patient is titrated up to the 'pain-free dose' with 4 hourly oral morphine solution and then changed to the same total 24 hour dose of M.S.T. tablets. For example:

if total 24 hour morphine in solution required = 60 mg

then M.S.T. dose = 30 mg b.d.

Phenazocine (Narphen)

Phenazocine tablets (5 mg) provide a useful alternative to morphine if the patient remains drowsy or nauseated on morphine despite adequate antiemetic dosages or when there is difficulty swallowing. It is best taken sublingually and can often be given 6 hourly. Phenazocine is also available as an injection.

Dipipanone in Diconal is in a fixed dose combination with cyclizine (an antiemetic). It often causes a dry mouth and drowsiness because the sedating cyclizine has to be increased as the analgesic dipipanone dose is raised. This combination drug is not usually suitable for flexible symptom control in terminal care.

Alternatives to oral analgesics

Suppositories

Few people accept that suppositories can be for anything other than bowel disorders. The mode of action must therefore be explained to patient and relatives. Suppositories provide an effective alternative in a patient unable to take oral drugs because of obstruction/dysphagia or persistent vomiting.

Oxycodone pectinate (30 mg or more): a useful, slow-release, effective analgesic which can be given 8 hourly; at time of writing only obtainable from Boots as a 'special' order.

Morphine suppositories: 10, 15, 20, 30 or 60 mg need to be given every 3–4 hours.

Injected opiates

Diamorphine injection, even in high doses, can be dissolved in 0.5 ml water and given subcutaneously, which is less painful than intramuscular injections. The dose must be given 4 hourly to keep the patient pain free.

N.B. 1 mg injected diamorphine = 3 mg morphine by mouth. Subcutaneous diamorphine infusion is useful for patients who are up and about at home. A continual infusion can be given by a steady-rate syringe driver, obtainable from most specialist units. Antiemetics are not always required with this route of administration.

Drugs to avoid for 24 hour pain control

Drug	Half-life (hours)	Reason
Pentazocine	2–4 (variable)	Unpredictable response to single dose Many patients become hallucinated Orally less potent than 2 Codis tablets Morphine antagonist and interferes with titration of an opiate for analgesia
Pethidine	$2\frac{1}{2}$	Needs to be given every 2 hours by injection to keep patient pain free Orally 50 mg pethidine is less potent than 2 Codis tablets
Dextromoramide (Palfium)	$1\frac{1}{2}$–2	Duration too short for regular use. It is a potent analgesic; for short-term use, e.g. during dressings
Methadone (Physeptone)	Up to 72	Accumulates to dangerous levels especially in elderly or frail patients
Buprenorphine (Temgesic)	8	Moderate analgesic Long term use not yet fully ascertained. Morphine antagonist in high doses
Dipipanone + Cyclizine in fixed combination (Diconal)	8	The fixed dose combination makes flexible symptom control impossible. Sedation, confusion and dry mouth can be problems
Dihydrocodeine (DF118)	4–6	Very constipating

BONE PAIN

Bony secondaries cause pain irrespective of their size.

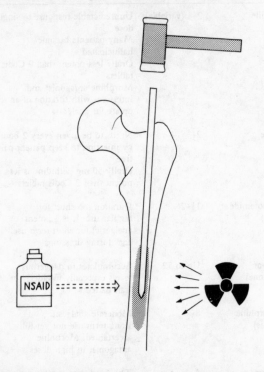

The NON-STEROIDAL ANTI-INFLAMMATORY DRUGS (NSAID) are the first-line analgesics for bone pain. Diflunisal, flurbiprofen, naproxen and other potent agents of this type are equally effective and the choice is fairly arbitrary. The drugs must be given regularly every 6–8 hours, often in high dose. They may take up to 3 weeks to be fully effective. Regular morphine may also be required to provide initial analgesia (see pages 16–17) and can sometimes be reduced or withdrawn when the NSAID is fully effective.

PALLIATIVE RADIOTHERAPY can be dramatically effective against local bony secondaries and it may produce complete analgesia after a single dose, even though the size of the lesion is unaltered.

If there is a serious risk of a pathological fracture, the bone should be ORTHOPAEDICALLY IMMOBILISED, either by internal pinning e.g. humerus or femur, or by external fixation, e.g. cervical collar.

**BONY SECONDARIES MAY
PRODUCE HYPERCALCAEMIA**

The hypercalcaemic syndrome includes vomiting, polydipsia with polyuria (which mimics diabetes) and resultant dehydration. Hypercalcaemia can also cause confusion.

In patients with bony secondaries, the serum calcium is not always raised, although they appear clinically hypercalcaemic. Either prednisolone (15–30 mg/day) or dexamethasone (2–4 mg/day) can be used to treat the syndrome.

COMMON SOURCES OF PAIN IN THE TERMINAL PATIENT

Generalised pains — intercurrent infections
osteomalacia
myalgic aches
post chemotherapy

At the site of tumour — infiltration of soft tissue or bone
cellulitis (don't forget anaerobes and candida)
nerve compression
post therapy — radiotherapy
chemotherapy
surgical scar neuralgia

Limb/back pains — bony secondaries
nerve compression
myofascial pains
cramps
pain in a paralysed limb from disuse
phantom limb
arthritis
lymphoedema
pressure sores

Headache — tension
migraine
raised intracranial pressure
associated with constipation

Abdomen — constipation
tumour deposits in organ especially hepatomegaly
cystitis
obstruction (any level)
dyspepsia

Chest — angina
         manifestation of anxiety
         tumour associated (see above)
         pleurisy
         chest wall (musculo-skeletal)
Ano-rectal pain — constipation and fissure
                           local tumour
Procedures causing pain: changing dressings
                                   moving/turning patient
                                   rectal procedures

ALL SYMPTOMS ARE MADE WORSE
BY FEAR, ANXIETY OR DEPRESSION

5

Nausea and vomiting

These are disabling symptoms in terminally ill patients and they should be relatively easy to control.

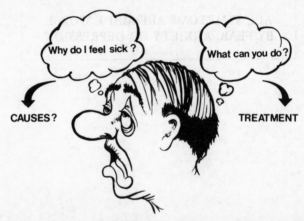

A search for the causes of nausea/vomiting is a prerequisite for logical therapy. Understanding how the various antiemetics act will lead to quicker control of these difficult symptoms. On the following two pages a schematic outline of the physio-pathology of nausea/vomiting is presented. The principle sites of action of antiemetic drugs are represented in a simplified form. It must, however, be emphasised that all the antiemetics listed have some central sedative effect which occurs in addition to their specified action. It must also be remembered that nausea/vomiting can occur in response to pain/fear and can become a conditioned reflex.

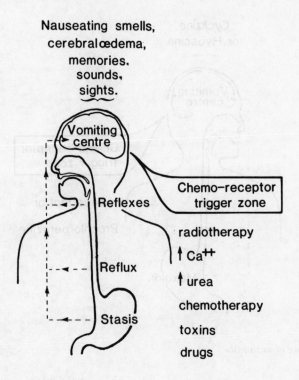

Physiology of vomiting

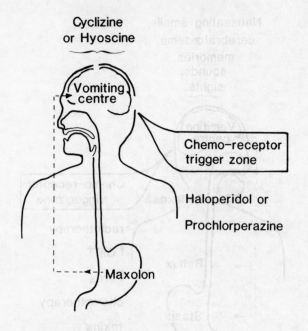

Choice of antiemetics

Ideal management is to treat the cause immediately and to give a single appropriate antiemetic to inhibit nausea and vomiting. However, pragmatic management is often required to relieve the distressing symptoms whilst the underlying cause is sought. Antiemetic drugs from each group should be added sequentially in adequate doses until the symptoms are controlled.

Metoclopramide 10–20 mg and haloperidol 0.5–2 mg can be given by slow intravenous injection and are rapidly effective. Prochlorperazine and other phenothiazines are available in suppository form. Steroids often help in a non-specific way, but they are vital if hypercalcaemia or raised intracranial pressure occur.

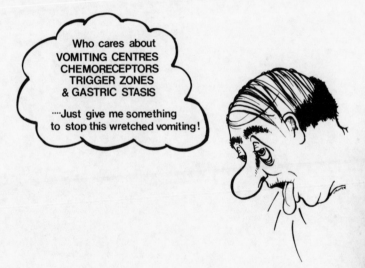

A suggested pragmatic regime to control acute vomiting is:

Metoclopramide 10 mg 8 hourly
    if symptoms persist ADD
Prochlorperazine 5 mg 8 hourly or haloperidol 0.5–5 mg 12 hourly
    if symptoms persist ADD
Cyclizine 50 mg 8 hourly
    if symptoms persist ADD
Prednisolone 10 mg or dexamethasone 0.5–2 mg 8 hourly.

The patient must be encouraged to be confident that the symptom can be controlled quickly. Hence the doctor/nurse must also have confidence in the therapeutic plans.

6

Constipation and its prevention

Normal bowel function is unrelated to the frequency of motion; it involves the passage of stools which are bulky yet having a consistency approximating that of toothpaste. People who are weak and dying usually consume less by mouth and exercise little so their chances of constipation are increased. They also often need drugs which may cause constipation as a side-effect.

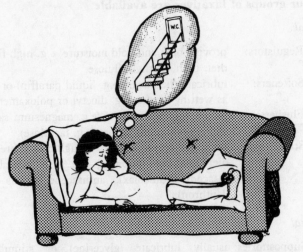

Is the patient more sedentary than is necessary? Is the patient over-sedated? Is the toilet accessible easily, so the patient can respond to the urge to defaecate? A commode or walking aid may help greatly.

Does the diet provide abundant fluid?

Does the diet provide adequate fibre?

If drugs such as dihydrocodeine, dextropropoxyphene, narcotics, tricyclics or phenothiazines are being prescribed, have you considered the need for laxatives as co-therapy?

Does the stool consistency approximate that of toothpaste?

**FAECAL SOILING OR COLICKY PAIN
IS AN INDICATION FOR RECTAL
EXAMINATION TO EXCLUDE IMPACTION**

If the rectum is empty consider whether the patient has high constipation (colon loaded on abdominal palpation). Ballooning of the rectum is usually caused by a mass in the colon.

Four groups of laxatives are available

Oral

Regulators:	provide bulk and hold moisture, e.g. high-fibre diet, bran, methylcellulose.
Softeners:	lubricate the bowel (e.g. liquid paraffin) or act as wetting agents (e.g. dioctyl or poloxamer).
Flushers:	act on the small bowel (e.g. magnesium salts) and non-absorbed sugars (e.g. lactulose).
Stimulants:	act on the colon. The best is high bulk (fibre) in diet but the following are also available: bisacodyl (dulcolax), anthracene (senna or danthron).

Rectal

Suppositories:	usually lubricate (glycerine) or stimulate chemically (bisacodyl or beogex).
Enemas:	lubricate (arachis oil or warm water) or stimulate (phosphate enema or sodium salts as micralax).

How do I choose a laxative?

Remember that appropriate food and drink are always the most important first step. Many weak patients do not experience thirst until clinically dehydrated, so they must be encouraged to take fluids every 1–2 hours.

In *simple constipation* combination mixtures are effective. They can be given as a single nightly dose or more frequently.

e.g.	*stool softener* +	*bowel stimulant*	
Dorbanex =	poloxamer +	danthron	(Dorbanex Forte is usually required as 5–20 ml nocte)
Normax =	dioctyl +	danthron	(2–6 caps, nocte or 1 cap, 4 hourly)

The dose of laxative should be increased until the stool is the consistency of toothpaste. An initial rapid evacuation is not an indication to stop therapy or the patient will swing back into constipation again.

Rectal procedures may be required initially to empty a loaded rectum/colon.

If the patient is too weak to push out a stool, gentle rectal evacuations may be required from time to time in addition to maintenance laxatives. Valium taken an hour or two before the procedure aids relaxation.

N.B. If the patient is at risk of intestinal obstruction from a narrowed bowel lumen, stool softeners must be started prophylactically and stimulant drugs which can cause colic should be avoided.

7

Intestinal obstruction

Intestinal obstruction (large bowel or ileum) will result in the patient having severe colicky abdominal pain. For the dying person a colostomy is a frightening procedure to which they will never have time to truly adapt.

Prophylactic measures must be taken early. A semi-liquid stool will be squeezed through a narrow atonic segment of bowel by adjacent peristalsis, but a hard mass of stool will cause obstruction.

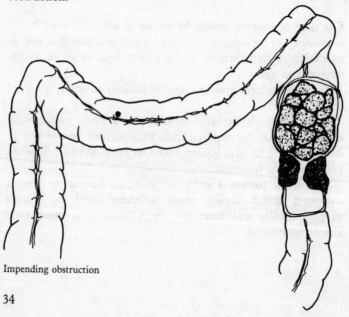

Impending obstruction

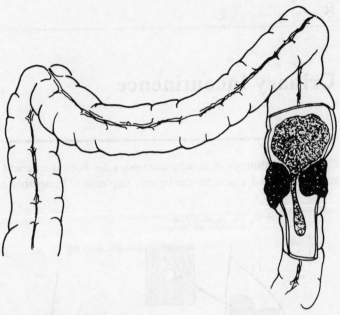

Softened stool

Very large doses of stool softener (dioctyl forte 8–12 tablets/day) must be given to encourage formation of semi-liquid stool.

If the patient develops colic, an antispasmodic, e.g. loperamide 2 mg 6-hourly can be given to control the symptom, whilst normal gastrointestinal function is sometimes encouraged by metoclopramide 10 mg 6–8 hourly.

8

Urinary incontinence

Urinary incontinence is equally distressing for both the patient and relatives and a catheter can be very unpleasant. Sympathetic

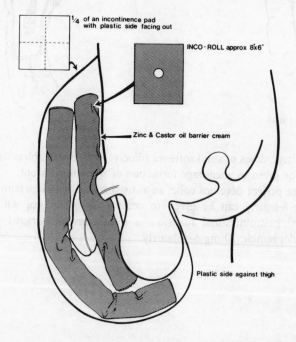

¼ of an incontinence pad with plastic side facing out

INCO - ROLL approx 8ʺx6ʺ

Zinc & Castor oil barrier cream

Plastic side against thigh

HOW TO AVOID A CATHETER IN THE LAST DAYS OF LIFE

nursing is essential and there are several important causes to be ruled out: constipation, urinary infection, neurological lesion (see p. 58), analgesic and other drugs causing oversedation, anterior vaginal wall prolapse in women.

HOW TO AVOID A CATHETER IN THE LAST DAYS OF LIFE

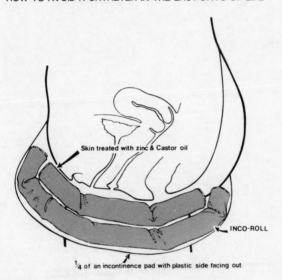

Skin treated with zinc & Castor oil

INCO-ROLL

¼ of an incontinence pad with plastic side facing out

A catheter can be avoided by using pads of absorbent wadding which can be cut in the required lengths from an incontinence roll and then placed snuggly inside firm fitting panties. This padding should be changed at least every 2 hours (when the bedbound patient is turned) and can easily be done by relatives. In the ambulant patient, firm fitting pads allow more mobility than a trailing catheter and bag. Skin should be protected with copious zinc and castor oil.

Many catheters leak so have no advantage if the motive is to keep the bedding dry! If a catheter is inserted, discuss it fairly with the patient so he or she does not feel bullied into accepting one and think beforehand whether you can save the patient the indignity of a catheter by using copious pads. If a catheter leaks, fit a smaller . . . not a size larger.

Incontinence aids — see Chapter 28.

9

Mouth care

Dehydration causes a dry mouth and halitosis.
Oral fluids must be encouraged in all patients able to swallow.
Malnutrition predisposes to many mouth problems.

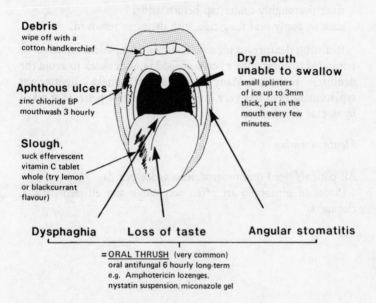

Debris
wipe off with a
cotton handkerchief

**Dry mouth
unable to swallow**
small splinters
of ice up to 3mm
thick, put in the
mouth every few
minutes.

Aphthous ulcers
zinc chloride BP
mouthwash 3 hourly

Slough,
suck effervescent
vitamin C tablet
whole (try lemon
or blackcurrant
flavour)

Dysphaghia   **Loss of taste**   **Angular stomatitis**

= <u>ORAL THRUSH</u> (very common)
oral antifungal 6 hourly long-term
e.g. Amphotericin lozenges,
nystatin suspension, miconazole gel

Alternatives to amphotericin are: nystatin suspension or
miconazole gel. A general oral antiseptic is Betadine mouth wash.

> ORAL THRUSH CAN CAUSE DISTORTION
> OF TASTE OR DYSPHAGIA LONG BEFORE
> MOUTH LESIONS ARE VISIBLE

Dentures

Dentures often hide oral thrush, even when they look clean. Standard denture cleaners do not destroy candida so the following procedure should be adopted when oral candida is suspected:

scrub the plate with a toothbrush;
sterilise overnight in a weak solution of bleach or by washing in boiling water;
rinse thoroughly under tap before using;
suck or apply oral fungicide with dentures removed.

Ill-fitting dentures can cause anorexia and patients need to be reminded to chew with a bolus of food in each cheek to avoid the dentures rocking. Many dentists will make lightweight replacement dentures very quickly for terminal patients if asked by doctor or relatives.

Mouth cleansing

All patients need oral toilet at least twice per day.
Pieces of pineapple are often acceptable and efficient mouth cleansers.

10

Anorexia

Common causes of anorexia in terminal patients are:

unpalatable presentation of food;

fatigue;   subclinical nausea;

constipation;   dehydration;

reactive — pain   mouth problems;

        anxiety

        discomfort;

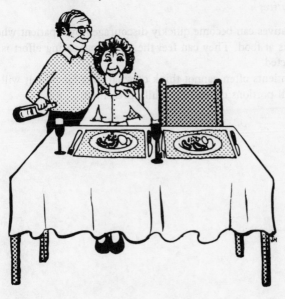

Measures which can help:

Sit the patient up for meals.

Sherry or other favoured appetiser given before the meal.

Improvement of physical comfort by ensuring that the patient has an empty bladder, bowel and a clean mouth as well as adequate analgesia before food is offered.

Fresh air from adequate ventilation will aid enjoyment of food.

Food must look appetising — small portions attractively presented are tempting.

Fluids are most important.

Eating is a social event normally — a person is more likely to enjoy eating in company than alone.

Sometimes glucocorticoids (e.g. prednisone 5 mg t.d.s.) are effective in anorexia due to malignancy, but this benefit is short lived. *am → mid pn. If given later may cause insomnia.*

Relatives

Relatives can become quickly discouraged by a patient who only picks at food. They can feel their personal caring effort is being rejected.

Patients often cannot think of what they fancy, but will enjoy small portions of food tastefully presented.

11

Dyspepsia

This is a common symptom in severely ill patients. It can contribute to anorexia and the choice of therapy must be based on careful assessment of possible causes.

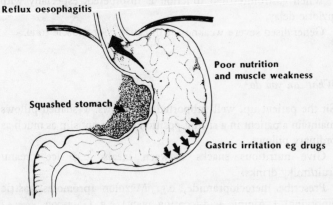

REMEMBER:

* Frequent small meals, with adequate fibre and nutrient content help most types of dyspepsia.

* Combination therapy is useful: in reflux — metoclopramide
+ alginic acid
in squashed stomach —
metoclopramide
+ defoaming antacid

* Alginic acid requires an acid medium to form a coating foam. It is therefore ineffective with defoaming agents, antacids and H_2 blockers, e.g. cimetidine.

* Cimetidine delays diazepam excretion.

Reflux oesophagitis

Who is at risk?

Supine patient and the patient who sits crumpled up in the bed.
   Patient with raised intra-abdominal pressure.
   When gastrointestinal function is disordered, especially with pyloric delay.
   Generalised severe weakness will cause poor muscle tone.

What can you do?

Sit the patient up, well supported on pillows. V-shaped pillows maintain a patient in a sitting position and do not slip as much as ordinary pillows.
   Give nutritious snacks between meals, e.g. ice cream/fruit/milky drinks.
   Prescribe metoclopramide, e.g. Maxolon (promotes gastric emptying) + Alginic acid (coating agent), e.g. Gaviscon.

Gastric irritation (Gastritis)

Who is at risk?

Many drugs are gastric irritants, e.g. aspirin, non-steroidal anti-inflammatory agents, steroids, iron, potassium, etc.
   Inadequate nutrition will predispose to dyspepsia and to peptic ulceration.

What can you do?

Food should be taken frequently especially before drug administration.

Drug regime should be reviewed to avoid irritant drugs, but if it cannot be altered H₂ blockers (e.g. cimetidine) should be considered. (Sucralfate (Antepsin) may be an alternative to H₂ blockers).

Simple antacids may be very effective if given freely.

Squashed stomach

Who is at risk?

Gastric function can be grossly deranged by physical distortion of the stomach, by tumour in the stomach wall itself or by external pressure from an enlarged liver or gross ascites (See figure on p. 43).

What can you do?

Food must be given in small frequent amounts because the gastric volume is reduced; 1–2 hours should be allowed between courses, e.g. soup/rest/small portion of meat and vegetables/rest/dessert, so the day becomes divided every 2 hours by some nutrition. Patients and relatives need help to understand that this alteration in routine is required because the gastric volume is small.

Metoclopramide promotes gastric emptying.

Defoaming antacids can also be useful as they reduce the volume of the gastric contents (e.g. Asilone, Polycrol, Altacite-Plus).

12

Hiccup

Protracted hiccup can be associated with:

* gastric distortion
* diaphragmatic irritation
* hepatomegaly
* uraemia
* aerophagy

DEHYDRATION, CONSTIPATION AND ANXIETY ALL MAKE HICCUP WORSE

Remember:

— PEPPERMINT WATER encourages eructation.
— DE-FOAMING AGENTS after meals reduce distension.
— METOCLOPRAMIDE improves gastric emptying.
— CHLORPROMAZINE 10–25 mg 6 hourly may help.

Traditional methods of pharyngeal counter-stimulation sometimes work, e.g. drinking from wrong side of cup, drinking with ears held covered.

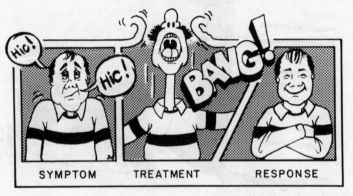

HOW · TO · CURE · HICCUPS

(or the 'Big Bang' theory)

SYMPTOM   TREATMENT   RESPONSE

13

Dyspnoea

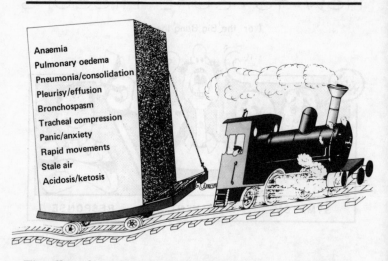

Anaemia
Pulmonary oedema
Pneumonia/consolidation
Pleurisy/effusion
Bronchospasm
Tracheal compression
Panic/anxiety
Rapid movements
Stale air
Acidosis/ketosis

The effort of breathing can sometimes be decreased by diuretics, bronchodilators and antibiotics. Patients should be nursed with the good lung uppermost to have the optimal ventilation-perfusion ratio. All movements should be undertaken calmly and slowly so that minimal effort is needed. A physiotherapist can teach relatives and the patient how to move together and can provide appropriate aids to facilitate mobility. Many patients feel better with free air circulating around their face; a free standing domestic electric fan or a hand-held battery operated fan is effective.

Any element of compression of the trachea or distortion of the parenchymal structure of the lung by tumour infiltrates, will often respond well to high dose steroids (see p. 58).

TREAT THE REVERSIBLE COMPONENT, THEN USE MORPHINE TO CONTROL RESIDUAL DYSPNOEA

Morphine, in doses above the analgesic dose for that patient will depress respiratory rate, but will not decrease tidal volume.

Oral morphine solution should be given 4-hourly. The dose should be titrated up until the symptom is controlled, i.e. when the patient is no longer distressingly breathless. Large regular doses of morphine (e.g. 100 mg 4 hourly) are often required.

Oxygen by mask provides only temporary relief. Tolerance develops rapidly, so the oxygen ceases to be effective. The mask is cold and sweaty and is a barrier to the patient communicating normally with the family. The emptying cylinder can frighten both relatives and patient, who become emotionally dependent on a relatively ineffective treatment. A nebuliser can be very helpful to provide bronchodilation or moisturized air when sputum is tenacious and difficult to expectorate.

14

Cough

The cough of resolving infection or clearing of airways is functionally useful whereas a persistent cough which is meaningless to the patient is exhausting. Sometimes the cause can be alleviated, e.g. cardiac failure, infection, pleural effusion, bronchospasm, etc. In terminal care symptomatic control is often a primary goal and difficult to attain. The following may be helpful:

* Linctus codeine
* Linctus methadone at night
* Palliative radiotherapy
* Morphine used in pain/dyspnoea will also suppress cough
* A nebuliser with bronchodilators will sometimes help enormously; even when bronchospasm is absent nebulised water or saline may be helpful if mucous is tenacious or airways feel dry and tickly.

15

Itch

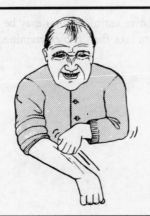

Problem	Plan
Is skin too dry?	Emollients, e.g. emulsifying ung.
Is there eczema or has scratching induced eczematisation?	Steroids topically Avoid woollen garments
Is it drug induced?	Review drug regime
Is the patient uraemic?	Try exposure to ultraviolet-B light, e.g. sun-lamp daily
Is there skin prickling on contact with water (= aquagenic pruritis)?	Wash quickly, dry with pre-warmed towels. Aspirin or antihistamines one hour before washing may help

The patient with generalised itching and normal looking skin (e.g. lymphoma) can be helped by

* keeping skin cool
* try $\frac{1}{2}$ per cent menthol in oily calamine applied hourly
* ung. emulsificans
* crotamiton (Eurax) may help
* sedative antihistamines are sometimes helpful, especially at night.

In liver failure sedative antihistamines may be effective and they are more pleasant to take than cholestyramine.

16

Pressure areas

The majority of patients at home are relatively mobile and not bedbound until the very end of their lives. Even when mobility is limited, any movement from bed to chair to commode will provide welcome relief to pressure areas.

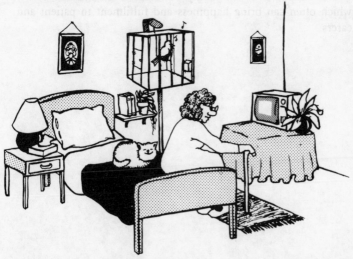

'Encourage activity and prevent pressure areas'

Bedsores are mechanically produced and the only effective prevention of them is the prevention of prolonged pressure on an area of skin. This entails frequent movement or turning of patients, which should be done at least every 2 hours. The ischaemic damage is not prevented by any systemic or topical preparations. Between nursing visits, relatives can often part-turn an immobile patient by moving supporting pillows from under one side of the patient's body to under the other side. However, every change of posture, however small, is helpful. Even stretching out for items beside the bed can lead to capillary perfusion in a pressure area.

The patient's best friend for preventing painful pressure areas is the gentle and competent community nurse who gives the family a number of practical hints and skills which will make regular movement possible in the most bedbound person. The nurse who tries to 'do it all herself' usually fails in a costly way and withholds from the family that close nursing involvement which often can bring happiness and fulfilment to patient and carers.

17

Fungating lesions

These are: unpleasant to look at,
often have offensive odour,
sometimes bleed,
can usually be controlled.

Action check list:

- Radiotherapist can often help
- Anaerobes cause odour:
  *Irrigate clean with 50 per cent EUSOL or NORMAL SALINE frequently
  *Flagyl may help temporarily (topically or systemically)
  *Gauze soaked in Betadine in liquid paraffin emulsion (equal parts) placed over the lesion
  *Room air smell absorbers[1]
  *Charcoal impregnated dry dressing[2]
  *Netelast will hold dressing in place without adhesive tape
  *Yoghurt dressings can be very effective
- Adequate ventilation and copious dressings help to avoid social embarrassment from

---

[1]Air smell absorbing sprays: Atmocol (on N.H.S. tariff) or Ozium.
Air smell absorbing filters: Electrically operated charcoal screens.
[2]Smell absorbing dressing covers: Nilodor or Denidor.

soiling and odour. A colostomy bag may be suitable for short-term coverage for special occasions, e.g. to go to shops/church, (N.B. Anaerobic if left too long).

When dressing changes are uncomfortable, dextromoramide (5–10 mg) ½-hour before the procedure will help. Alternatively 50 per cent nitrous oxide in oxygen can be administered during the procedure.

MODERN RADIOTHERAPY OFTEN CAN CONTROL FUNGATING LESIONS

18

Bleeding lesions

For example, haemoptysis and uterine or rectal malignancies.

Palliative radiotherapy may decrease blood loss or discharge from many malignant lesions.

Rectal steroid preparations sometimes decrease unpleasant discharge from malignant lesions in the rectum.

19

Compression syndromes

* Nerve compression
* Tracheal compression
* Superior venacaval obstruction
* Raised intracranial pressure
* Lymphatic/venous compression
* Pharyngeal/oesophageal pressure
* Pulmonary infiltration by tumour

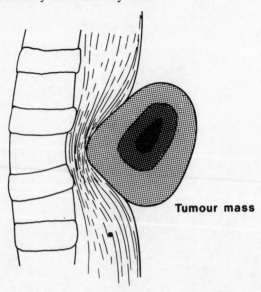

Tumour mass

In all these syndromes the tumour is compressing an adjacent structure, thereby causing distressing symptoms. Around the tumour mass there is an area of oedema or hyperaemia and this can be shrunk by high dose steroids or by palliative radiotherapy.

Suggested regime

1. *Steroids.* Dexamethasone must be started in high dose to gain the maximum benefit.

   Initial dose = dexamethasone 4 mg 6 hourly until the symptom is controlled (usually under 1 week) then decrease gradually to a maintenance dose, usually about 2 mg/day.

2. *Consult radiotherapist/oncologist* early because a single dose of palliative radiotherapy may suffice and will not cause any distressing side-effects.

Specific measures for specific problems

Dysphagia — semi-liquid nutrition, especially cold foods, e.g. ice-cream.

Dyspnoea — see Chapter 13.

Lymphoedema — external compression either with an elasticated bandage or an inflatable intermittent-compression sleeve (obtainable from specialist centres and several surgical units or physiotherapy departments).

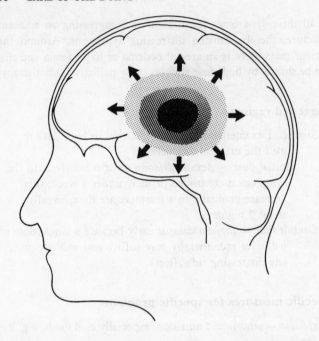

Headache of raised intracranial pressure — codeine phosphate is the analgesic of choice, doses of 60 mg 4 hourly can be given by mouth or, if the patient is vomiting, by subcutaneous injection. Morphine is not a suitable analgesic; it may in fact worsen the headache.

Patients should be nursed in the sitting position and potent diuretics may give additional short-lived relief.

20

Confusion

* Visual messages can be confused with memories:
  e.g. a visitor may be perceived as someone else.
* Sounds can be misinterpreted:
  e.g. voices/television may be felt to be threats.
* Touch or bedclothes may be perceived as restraints:
  e.g. 'let me go . . . release me . . .'
* Fears may surface as accusations against carers:
  e.g. 'that nurse is stealing my money'.

The jumbled messages from many sensory pathways cause turmoil in the confused persons mind.

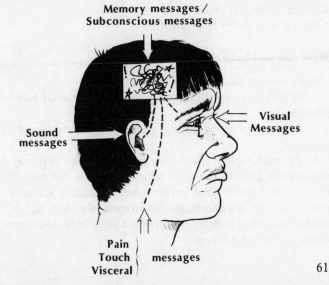

Memory messages /
Subconscious messages

Visual
Messages

Sound
messages

Pain
Touch
Visceral
} messages

Confusion can be precipitated by discomfort

e.g. full bladder
bedding badly made
pruritis
strange surroundings
background strange noise
poor lighting.

Predisposing factors to confusion

Drug toxicity — analgesics
phenothiazines
tricyclics } Too high dose or
pentazocine   impaired clearance
hypnotics/tranquillisers

Infection, e.g. pneumonia (may be apyrexial)
Anoxia (especially in mild cardiac failure).
Biochemical — hypercalcaemia
hypoglycaemia
hepatic/renal failure
Cerebral damage (C.V.A.)
Cerebral secondaries or primary

How can you help the confused patient?

1. By looking for the causative factor(s).

2. By nursing in a well-lit familiar place with familiar people if possible.

3. By not arguing or getting upset about the misinterpreted messages.

4. By encouraging relatives/carers to find the best way to reassure the troubled mind — sometimes gentle but reassuring touch, sometimes a quiet environment, sometimes a return to more familiar surroundings, sometimes the sharing of a reassuring mutual memory, sometimes a night-light, sometimes a favourite food or drink, etc.

5. By avoiding making things worse by being quick to sedate. Many sedative drugs can themselves cause confusion.

6. By remembering that confusion is often temporary and it often resolves when the triggers or causes are removed or modified.

**A GENTLE REASSURING TOUCH
CAN CALM A PATIENT BETTER
THAN WORDS OR DRUGS**

Excessive drowsiness may be due to fatigue, but the other possible causes are the same as those which predispose to confusion.

21

Insomnia

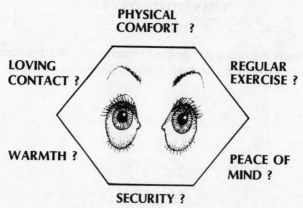

PHYSICAL
COMFORT ?

LOVING
CONTACT ?

REGULAR
EXERCISE ?

WARMTH ?

PEACE OF
MIND ?

SECURITY ?

The six facets of insomnia

When you cannot sleep you are usually separated from one or more of these facets. People who are dying are often lonely or weak or in pain or anxious — ideal management is to alleviate the causes.

The doctor or nurse is not always the best person to deal with all aspects of insomnia, but should make an accurate assessment and can suggest alternatives: a spouse, child, parent, solicitor, friend, employer, clergyman or social worker may be the right person to help with one or more of the facets of insomnia. A sympathetic listener last thing at night is invaluable.

Hypnotics may occasionally be necessary as a second-line approach and they should not be withheld if insomnia is worrying the patient — but neither should they be imposed if the patient is content with little sleep; this could be physiological.

* Short acting hypnotics
{
Temazepam (20–60 mg)
or
Chlormethiazole (2 capsules or 10 ml syrup)
}

* Long acting hypnotics are really just tranquillisers

* Major tranquillisers (e.g. chlorpromazine) are often useful as sedatives, co-analgesics and antiemetics

*Sometimes depression needs treatment pharmacologically

22

Weakness

Weakness is demoralising for the patient and family. Both need encouragement to maintain their roles within the home even as physical independence wanes. Fatigue from enjoyment is healthy and will not shorten a person's life; fatigue from boredom can result in depression.

Physiotherapists have much to offer and can encourage mobility by teaching efficient ways of moving and providing suitable aids to increase the patient's independence.

Why is the patient so weak?

Are drugs causing sedation?
Is the patient anaemic? Would a blood transfusion help?
Is there occult infection?
Is the patient uraemic?
Are neurological secondaries present?
Is the patient malnourished?
Is the patient dehydrated/ketotic? Frequent small amounts to drink are easier to take, e.g. $\frac{1}{4}$ cup of fluid every $\frac{1}{2}$ hour.
STEROIDS (prednisolone 10 mg 8 hourly or dexamethasone 0.5 mg 8 hourly) can give a general feeling of well-being, but the effect is relatively short-lived. In higher doses steroids can give a dramatic temporary improvement in a patient who wishes to participate in a special event, e.g. a family anniversary.

23

The patient in the family

Care of a dying relative at home is bound to modify attitudes within the home to a certain extent. However, it is important for all members of the household to keep their life-styles as normal as possible and to avoid making the ill person into an invalid before dependency is really necessary. Involvement in household decisions and family affairs is important for all members if self-respect is to be maintained.

Good symptom control should enable most patients to continue pursuits previously enjoyed (e.g. entertainments, parks, sport, shopping, etc) and maintenance of mobility will help the individual feel independent. An excellent morale booster, even for the bed-bound, is attention from a hairdresser or barber. The ambulant will find self respect in clothes which flatter. Disfiguring lesions can often be disguised satisfactorily by wigs, loose clothing and use of cosmetics.

The children in a family feel most secure when they are involved in the care of the dying person, particularly if their school, friendship and activity routines can be maintained. When a child is the patient there is a great danger that the whole household will alter their routines to provide a special environment for the ill child alone, forgetting that the other children need to be involved and feel loved. A similar situation can arise with elderly or demanding patients who can dominate the entire household and disrupt family life to an unacceptable extent.

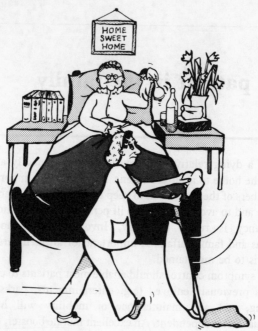

Being a carer can be tough

The process of caring for a dying relative is preparation for bereavement provided the carers feel involved and grow to realise that they are providing the best possible care. This confidence in the home can only develop if the professionals frequently voice their approval of the home care and anticipate stresses.

> ## WHEN RELATIVES ARE EXHAUSTED OR WORN THEY MAY NEED ENCOURAGEMENT AND THEY MAY NEED A BREAK

A few days for the patient in hospice or hospital or special home should be planned before the family ask for it. They must know that periodic relief is available before the strain gets too great. Primary physicians and nurses must fight for this facility for their patients in centres where it does not exist. Even when relatives refuse the offer of relief they should be aware that it exists (provided it does!).

Remember too that help with laundry, shopping, housework or sitters (day or night) often makes it possible for relatives to go on coping. Church or voluntary helpers will often be willing to give such aid if nurse, doctor or social worker suggest appropriate contacts.

> ## DO YOU KNOW THE NAMES AND ADDRESSES OF LOCAL ORGANISATIONS WHO WILL HELP TO STRENGTHEN HOME CARE IN YOUR AREA?

24

As death approaches

Relatives facing loss find the last hours hard to bear. They can gain comfort from being involved in caring and they need encouragement to touch, hold and talk to the dying person, even if he or she does not appear to register those around. Hearing is the last sense to be lost. It is never too late for a relative to confide in the dying person or apologise for past grievances.

```
THE UNRESPONSIVE PATIENT
CAN OFTEN STILL HEAR
```

Relatives also need reassurance that death should be peaceful and that breathing will gradually cease. They need reassurance that nothing needs to be done urgently after death, but they must be provided with free accesss to familiar nursing and medical advice.

Inability to swallow

If the patient becomes unable to swallow, analgesics and antiemetics must be continued at the equivalent dose to avoid the patient being re-aroused by pain or other distressing symptoms. A dry mouth can be kept moist with slithers of ice (see p. 39).

The following drugs are available as suppositories

Oxycodone pectinate	— insert 8 hourly
Morphine sulphate	— insert 4 hourly
Prochlorperazine	— insert 8 hourly
Chlorpromazine	— insert 8 hourly
Diazepam	— insert 12 hourly

If injections have to be given, the subcutaneous route is less painful than intramuscular injections and equally effective in most cases. The following drugs are useful subcutaneously:

Diamorphine

Haloperidol

Hyoscine

Terbutylene

Rectal tubes to deliver rapidly Diazepam in standard dose rapidly are now available for easy control of convulsions by relatives or non-medical carers.

Death rattle

A death rattle is due to secretions accumulating. Subcutaneous HYOSCINE in doses of 0.4–0.6 mg will diminish secretions if given early and can thereby abolish death rattle.

Hyoscine is also useful in a crisis, e.g. massive pulmonary embolus or haemorrhage since it provides a small degree of retrograde amnesia, so, if the patient recovers, the memory of the event is slightly blunted. Hyoscine combined with diamorphine is often a good combination under these circumstances.

25

Grief

HELPING THE GRIEVING

To understand and be available is the best primary treatment.

"Grief is like being on the edge of a volcano - a feeling as if something terrible is about to happen."
(Murray-Parkes, 1981)

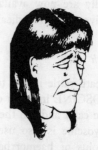

Grieving people have to re-live events over and over again....
often angry with themselves/ others ....this is a normal way of showing how much the lost one is loved........
'I will never forget.........

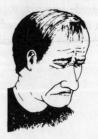

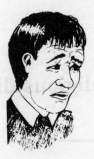

The physical experiences associated with grief can be very frightening............

Bereavement is not an event it is a process which should start before the loved one dies and has well defined physiology (and pathology)

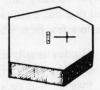

* Involving relatives in care of the dying helps to prepare for the loss.
* An opportunity to say good-bye to the dead person helps.
* Familiarity with normal grief will help the clinician recognise pathological deviation.
* Grief is a maturing experience, but it is hard to bear.
* Sometimes people need encouragement (permission) to stop grieving and to start to live again themselves.
* Many clergy, social workers and counsellors are able to help. The mix of physical, emotional, social and spiritual problems in grief often means that no one person is sufficient, even for those with a deep and secure faith.
* Bereavement is normal, it should not be made into a disease without very good clinical reasons.

26

Religious differences

Death, dying and grieving generate very different responses in different cultures and religious groups. The behaviours are so varied that this handbook cannot do justice to the topic except to point to a few facts which may be helpful:

* Hindus usually have their holy book (Bhagvad Gita) read to them by priest or family while they are dying and a thread may be tied round the neck or wrist to facilitate prayer. Many Hindus are very particular about who touches the body after death. No religious prohibition against autopsy.
* Moslems should be facing Mecca when they die while family members whisper prayers into the dying person's ear. The Koran is their holy book. According to Islamic Law the body must be buried within 24 hours and the body should never be cut or harmed after death. No cremations.
* Sikhs recite/read from the Gura Grant Sahab as death approaches. The whole family normally gathers around the death bed for prayer. Autopsy is not prohibited.
* Jews have strict codes of conduct about who may touch the body after death.

Grief experiences are enormously varied, from the silent or private British type of mourning in which restrained behaviour is admired to the strong displays of emotion which are expected in many Asian cultures[1].

---

[1]Fuller details in Henly A. Asian Patients in Hospital and at Home. King Edward Hospital Fund for London 1979.

The doctor or nurse who cares for dying people cannot remember all the ethnic differences, but he/she can be sensitive to key issues like

— who should be present at the death bed?
— how urgent is the burial procedure?
— is autopsy prohibited?
— is grief following normal patterns for the culture?

Most families will guide the clinician if given the opportunity to express ethnic and religious differences.

27

What to do after an expected death (UK)

Before Registration

* If eyes are to be donated, contact nearest eye hospital. If the body is to be used for research or teaching purposes, contact the Medical School with whom the patient made the arrangements. (See below for funeral arrangements).
* Report to the coroner/procurator fiscal (Scotland) if the death was caused by an industrial disease, e.g. asbestosis, cadmium poisoning, pneumoconiosis. An inquest will then be held.
* In the event of delay for the coroner's hearing, a letter confirming the fact of death can be obtained from the coroner's office. This may be needed for social security and insurance benefit purposes.
* A death referred to the coroner cannot be registered until the coroner/procurator fiscal has given a note of authority to the registrar.
* To move the body abroad permission must be obtained in every case from the coroner/procurator fiscal. This applies to moving a body from England and Wales to Scotland.

Registration

* Death must normally be registered within 5 days. A funeral cannot be arranged until the funeral director has a certificate for disposal from the registrar.

* The following are required to register a death:
  The medical certificate of the cause of death.
  The dead person's NHS medical card, if available.
  Any war pension book or other non-DHSS pension book
  (e.g. NHS pension) if available.
* The registrar will require to know the following
  information:
  date and place of birth;
  dead person's usual address;
  full names and surname and maiden name;
  dead person's date of birth and place of birth;
  marital status and how often married and to whom;
  dead person's occupation or occupation of husband(s);
  details of parentage may be required;
  any social security allowances or pension that were being
  received;
  if the dead person was married, the date of birth of the
  surviving spouse;
  name and address of patient's general practitioner.
* The certificate of registration of death must be taken to the
  local DHSS office to claim the death grant and/or widow's
  pension.
* Additional death certificates may be required for the will.
  These cost more if requested more than 7 days after
  registration[1].

Funeral

If the body is to be given for medical/teaching purposes, the
medical school will pay for a simple funeral and claim the death
grant. The body used for teaching must be buried or cremated
within 2 years. Bodies are refused if a post mortem has been held
or if any organs have been removed. Private arrangements can be

---

[1]In Scotland specific death certificates are required for each insurance policy.
The registrar needs to know the names of the proposer, life assured, payee and
insurance company.

made with a Minister of Religion for a remembrance service in lieu of a funeral/cremation service.

* Claims for financial help with a funeral must be made to the local social security offices before making any arrangements. Possible sources of additional financial help are:
  — if the next of kin gets supplementary benefit or works part-time, earnings being just above the supplementary benefit level;
  — from the dead person's employer/trade union;
  — an advance on insurance monies will be paid when probate is granted;
  — tax refund for the dead person (contact the tax office);
  — dead person's savings, on production of evidence of death.

* The local council (or area health authority for a death in hospital) will bury or cremate if no other arrangements can be made, but they will not pay for funeral arrangements made privately.

* Burial space or lair (Scotland) may have been bought already. This may be mentioned in the will. A faculty document is issued when a space is bought in a parish graveyard. A deed of grant or lair certificate (Scotland) is issued when a grave space has been bought in a cemetery (usually non-denominational).

The will

* A will appoints one or more people to be executors. The executor may gain a grant of probate or document of confirmation (Scotland) to dispose of the estate in accordance with the will.

* If there is no will, letters of administration or confirmation (Scotland) must be obtained from the probate/registry/sheriff clerk (Scotland). This can be done through a solicitor/lawyer (Scotland).

28

Aids

Incontinence aids: usually available through district nursing or hospital supplies:

Commode

Bed pan/urinal (wide necked 1 litre glass fruit jars are excellent substitutes for male urinals)

Disposable pants — elasticated (some patients find these easier to use with pads than incontinence pants) — can be re-used a few times.

Incontinence pants (Kanga, Maxi-plus, Hygi, Slipad, etc)

Disposable pads for stretch pants

Disposable pads for incontinence pants

Incontinence pads (for a chair etc)

Plastic drawsheet

Kylie drawsheets

Mobility aids: usually obtained through occupational therapy departments:

Walking aids — Zimmer, tripod, etc

Wheel chair and wheel chair cushion (ring, Spenco, etc)

Raised toilet seat

Geriatric chair

Rope ladder

Aids to nurse the bed-bound patient at home: usually obtained from district nursing services:

Hospital bed
Backrest
Monkey pole
Hoist
Ripple mattress/Spenco mattress
Sheepskins/Decubicare heel and elbow pads

Other aids to improve patient comfort: obtained from occupational or physiotherapy department:

Food liquidiser
Feeding cup
Leg rest
Intermittent-compression limb sleeve
Electric heated pad
Nebuliser
Deodoriser (electrically-driven charcoal filter screen)

Items which usually have to be purchased:

Transcutaneous nerve stimulator (may be obtainable from some pain clinics)
Fan (large electric or hand-held battery operated)
Delta V-shaped pillow
Quilt
Bed table

29

Topics for discussion

1. Mrs Jones (52) has disseminated carcinoma of the breast with multiple bony secondaries but she has remained ambulant and comfortable on slow-release morphine 60 mg b.d. (M.S.T.—60 b.d.) with a non-steroidal anti-inflammatory drug and laxative/stool softener mixture. Discuss:

   (a) Why she does not need an anti-emetic?   (Chapter 5)
   (b) What you would do if she developed anorexia?
                                                (Chapter 10)
   (c) Your course of action if she started to have colicy abdominal pain?   (Chapters 4, 6 and 7)
   (d) How would you manage a frozen shoulder if one starts developing?   (Chapter 4)

2. It is not uncommon for the family of a dying patient to prefer to cope alone at home without even a district nurse being in attendance. Discuss why this should be so
                                                (Chapters 1, 2 and 23)

3. I can't taste a thing doctor . . . it (my taste) will return won't it? (patient with carcinoma of lung).
   Discuss your management of this problem
                                                (Chapters 9 and 10)

4. Draw a clock face similar to the one on page 8 and record the duration of action for your first choice of:

   (a) oral narcotic in dying patients   (Chapter 4)
   (b) antiemetic in dying patients   (Chapter 5)

(c) slow-release morphine   (Chapter 4)

(d) favourite hypnotic   (Chapter 21)

5. I always tell my patients their diagnosis as soon as it is confirmed. (surgeon with special interest in breast disease). Discuss this comment   (Chapters 2 and 23)

6. Intern on telephone to specialist: Mrs James, the lady with carcinomatosis of uncertain origin, has been very aggresive and difficult since you admitted her last night ... her relatives are very upset because she has never been like this before and chlorpromazine 200 mg at 1 am didn't seem to help ...

What advice or help should the doctor in charge give the intern whose predicament also reflects the frustrations of the nursing staff?   (Chapter 20)

7. You are caring for an elderly lady who is ambulant but mildly demented and living with a daughter who has decided to keep her mother at home for the final illness (Ca. lung). The two women are alone in the house without close relatives near by. The old lady has taken a variety of drugs for some months. Create a check-list of items which you would expect any caring doctor or nurse to consider

(Chapters 1, 3 and 23)

8. Anxious patient with carcinoma of lung: I haven't had my bowels open for three days.

Patient's wife: But you haven't been eating my dear so that is hardly surprising.

How would (nurse or doctor) respond to this conversation?

(Chapters 6 and 10).

9. 'A doctor must always lead the team of people who care for dying patients.' This was stated by a well known specialist in terminal care. Encourage your group to discuss the comment in the light of patients' needs (Chapters 1 and 23)

10. Sunday morning, 9 am, the telephone rings in Dr Smith's house. A district nurse feels that Mrs K needs catheterisation because her relatives cannot cope with any more

soggy linen. Mrs K (58 years) is bed-bound with multiple sclerosis and dysphagia, she is unlikely to live more than a few more days.

What should be done?   (Chapters 8, 9, 16 and 24)

11. The meaningless persistent cough of infiltrating malignant lung disease is often matched by the gradual onset of terrifying dyspnoea. Create a list of principles and practices to reflect your group's approach to these problems.

(Chapters 13, 14 and 19)

12. 'Death has no sting for those with a strong faith but it is the "end" for the pragmatic majority . . . you deceive yourself if you claim that you can give hope in a situation where to die is the only option.' This view is sometimes expressed by people who work on the touch-lines of terminal care. How would your group reply?   (Chapters 1, 2 and 25)

13. Miss P. R. has generalised pruritus and dysphagia due to gastric carcinoma with liver secondaries. She is now having difficulty in taking any medication by mouth yet needs narcotics, antiemetics, etc. Your partner says 'for goodness sake get her into hospital . . . just say that she has to go'. Discuss your management options for the closing days of her life.   (Chapters 4, 9, 11, 15 and 19)